LOOK AFTER YOURSELF

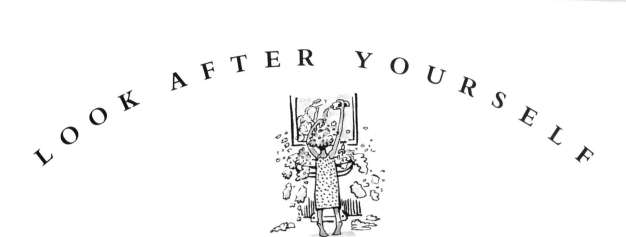

Keep Clean!

Anne Qualter & John Quinn

(4)
613.4

Wayland

Other titles in series

Stay Fit!
Healthy Food
Stay Safe!

Series editor: Catherine Baxter
Design: Loraine Hayes Design
Illustration: John Yates/Alan Preston

First published in 1993 by
Wayland (Publishers) Limited
61 Western Road, Hove
East Sussex, BN3 1JD, England
© Copyright 1993 Wayland (Publishers) Ltd.

British Library Cataloguing in Publication Data
Quinn, John
Keep Clean! – (Look After Yourself Series)
I. Title II. Qualter, Anne III. Series
613
ISBN 0 7502 0872 4

Typeset by Dorchester Typesetting Group
Limited
Printed and bound by B.P.C.C. Paulton Books

Photographs by permission of: Bruce
Coleman 13 (Alain Compost); Chapel
Studios 4, 5, 7, 9, 17, 18, 20, 22 (bottom),
23, 24; DLP Photo Library 13, 24; Eye
Ubiquitous 18; Life File 25; Reflections
cover, 8; Science Photo Library 10 (top,
CNRI/bottom left, Claude Nuridsany &
Marie Perennou/bottom right, EM Unit,
University of Southampton), 19 (Simon
Fraser), 21 (Dr Jeremy Burgess), 28
(James Stevenson); Skjold 29; Wayland
Picture Library 12, 15, 22 (top), 26.

Contents

Introduction

Good morning!

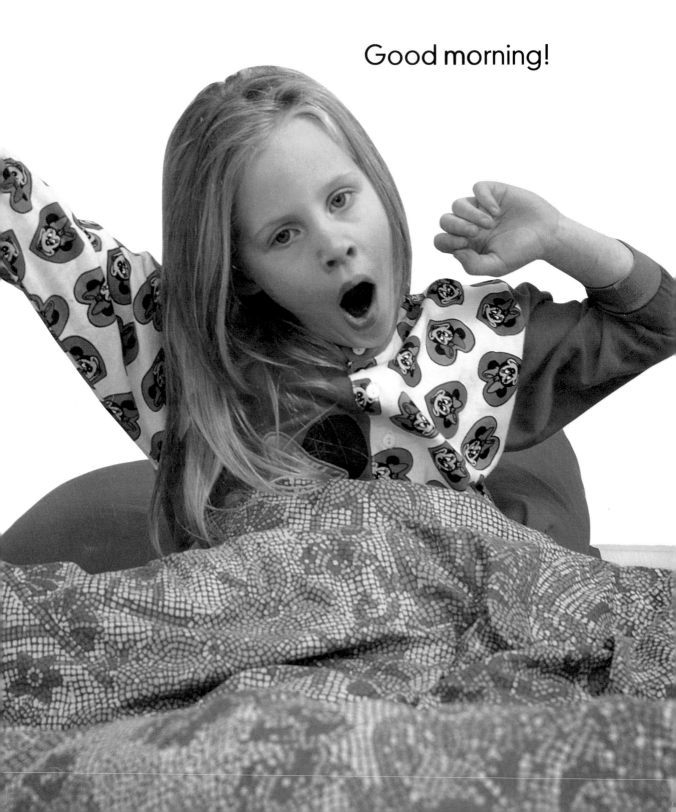

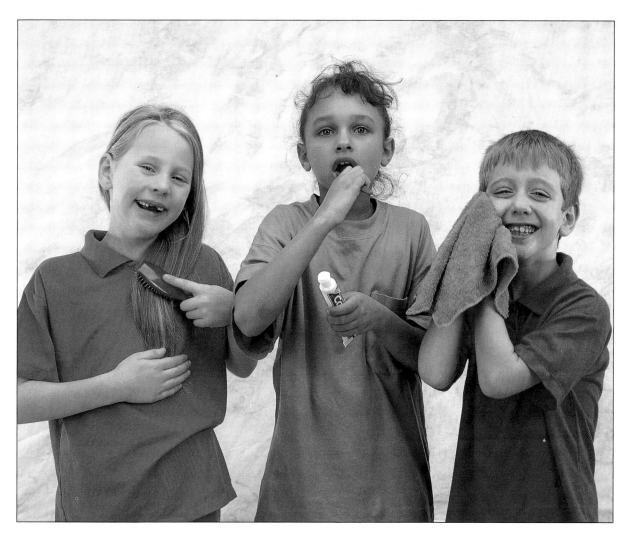

What do you do in the morning?

Brush your hair.

Brush your teeth.

Wash your face.

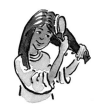

Why do you do all these things? You need to keep clean because it helps you to stay healthy.

Your skin

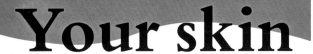

Your skin protects you. It stops harmful things getting to your insides. It separates your insides from the outside world. You have to look after your skin to keep it healthy.

This is a diagram of your skin.

sweat pore

hair

top layer of skin

lower layer of skin

oil gland

sweat gland

blood vessel

Very small things called germs are all around us. Most germs don't do us any harm, but some could if they got the chance. You have germs all over your skin. Washing gets rid of most of them.

Look at your skin under a hand lens. ▶

You can see lots of little lines, hairs and small marks where the hairs grow. You can't see germs because they are so very tiny.

Soap and water

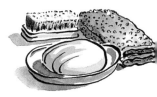

Why do we need soap?

Press your thumb against some clear plastic. Hold the plastic up to the light. What can you see?

Your skin makes oil. Your thumbprint is the greasy mark left by the oil. The oil keeps your skin waterproof. But it also means that dirt sticks to your skin. Soap sticks water and grease together. This means you can splash off dirt by washing.

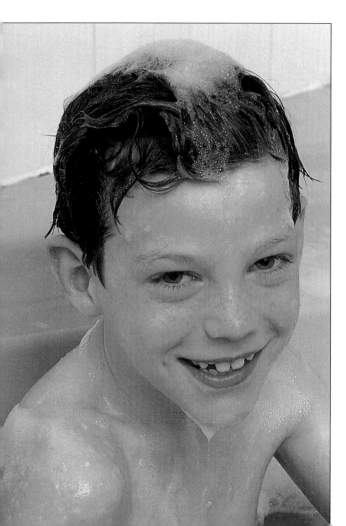

WOW!
Soap was first made in the Middle East more than 5000 years ago. It was made from a mixture of fat and the ashes from fires.

Grease a plate with margarine. Drip some water on to it. The water rolls off, and the plate stays greasy. Now drip water mixed with washing-up liquid on to the plate. What happens? ▼

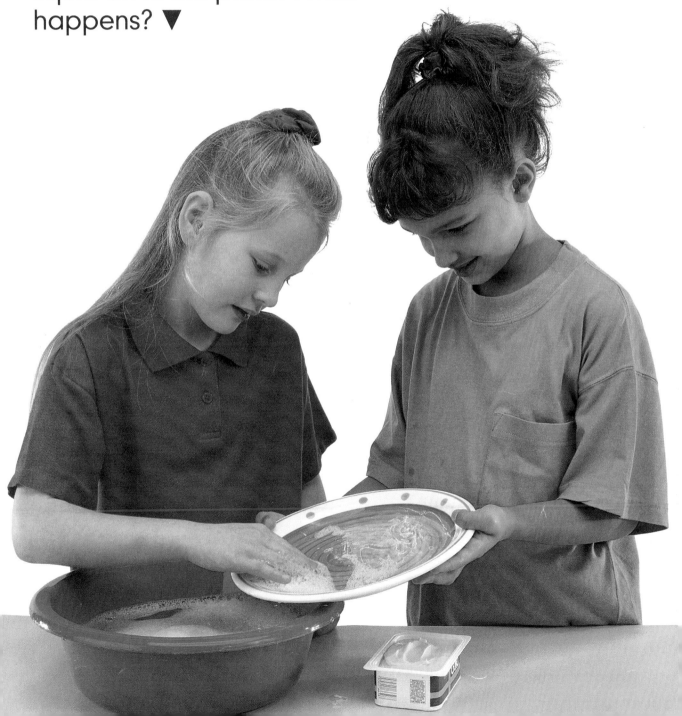

Germs

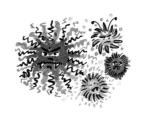

If you don't keep your skin clean, germs build up and you begin to smell. Sometimes small cuts or scratches can get germs in them. Then more germs grow and cause infection.

There are three types of germs – fungi, bacteria and viruses. They are so small that, normally, you can't see them. This is what they look like under a microscope. False colour has been added to help you see the shapes.

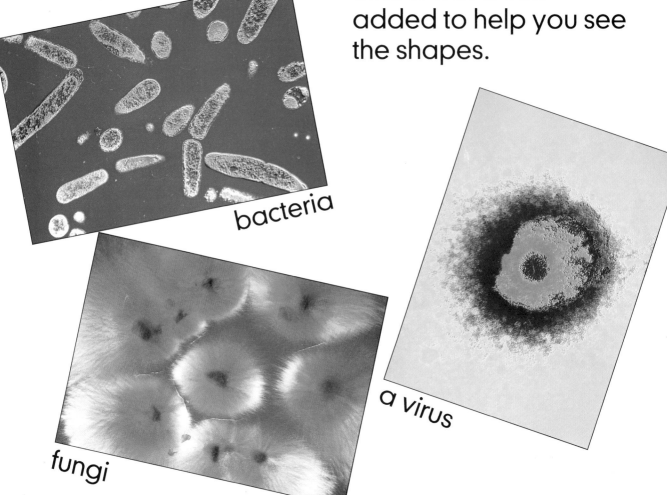

bacteria

fungi

a virus

How to keep clean

Always use soap
and water.

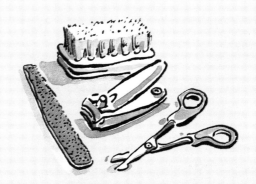

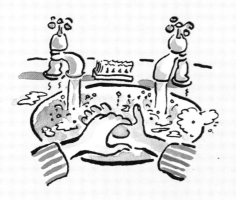

Keep your nails
short and use a nail
brush.

Bath or shower
frequently.

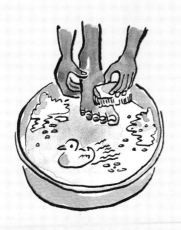

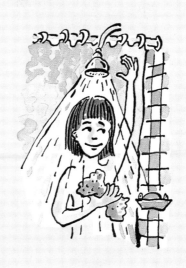

Change your socks
and wash your feet
regularly.

Your teeth

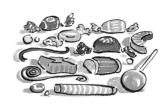

Have you noticed that your teeth feel rough sometimes? Inside your mouth are bacteria called plaque. Plaque grows very well if you eat a lot of sweet things. It can damage the smooth, shiny, white covering on your teeth, and let bacteria in which make your teeth rot. This can be very painful. ▼

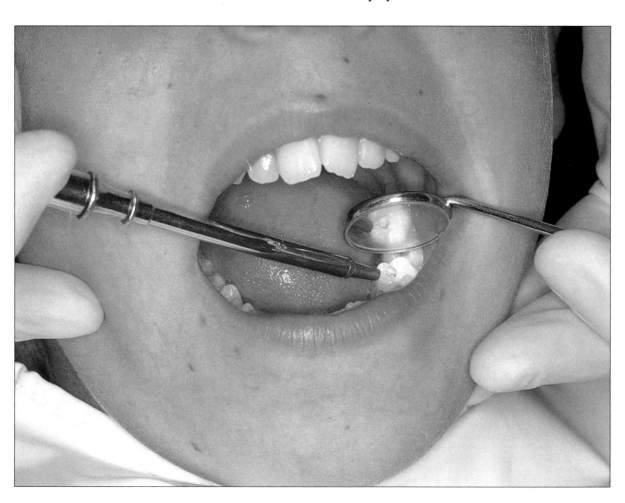

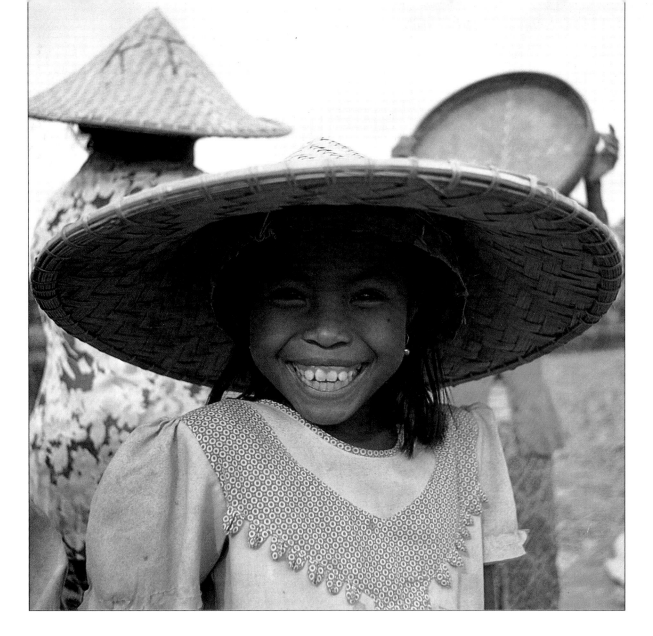

Eating fewer sweet ▲ things will help you not to get plaque. In some parts of the world, people have healthy teeth – this is because they don't eat many sweet things.

WOW!
Sharks grow new teeth throughout their lives. We only get two sets.

Clean teeth

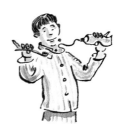

Brushing your teeth keeps plaque down and protects teeth and gums. You should brush your teeth at bed-time and after eating – not before.

This is how you should brush your teeth. ▼

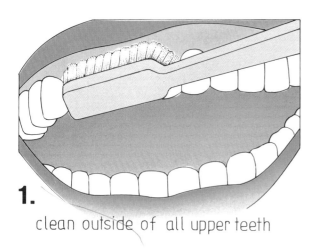

1. clean outside of all upper teeth

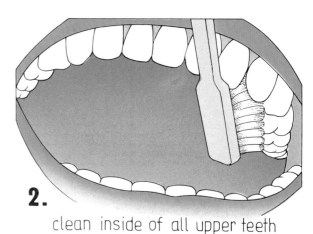

2. clean inside of all upper teeth

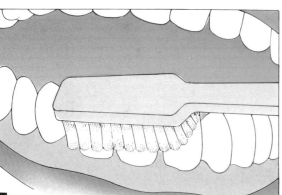

3. clean outside and inside of all lower teeth

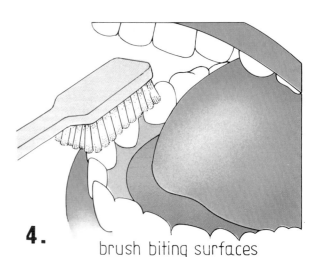

4. brush biting surfaces

If you want to make sure that you are brushing your teeth properly, buy disclosing tablets at the chemist's. When you suck one, it dyes the plaque. Try it and see.

After you have brushed your teeth, suck another tablet and you can see whether you have done it properly. There should be no dye on your teeth. If there is, brush some more!

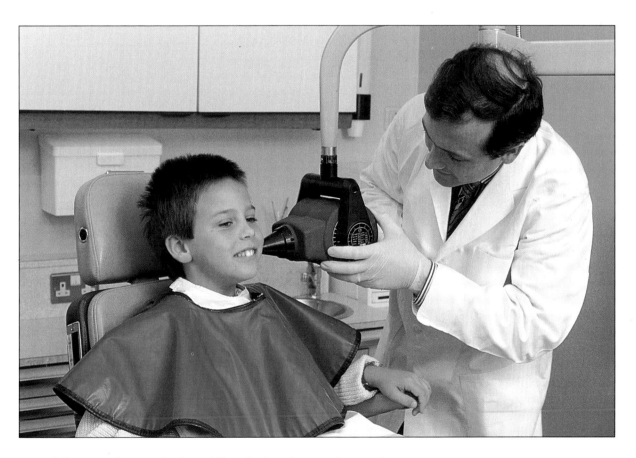

▲ You should still visit the dentist regularly to make sure your teeth and gums are healthy.

Cuts

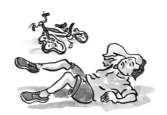

A cut in your skin can let germs in. But your blood comes to the rescue. When the blood comes out of the cut it meets the air and gets thicker. Eventually, it makes a scab.

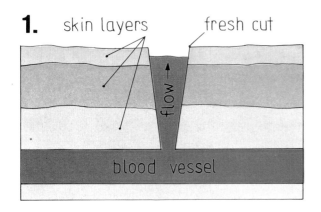

1. skin layers   fresh cut
flow →
blood vessel

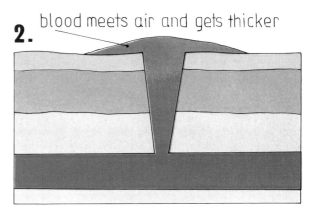

2. blood meets air and gets thicker

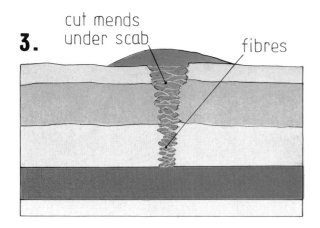

3. cut mends under scab   fibres

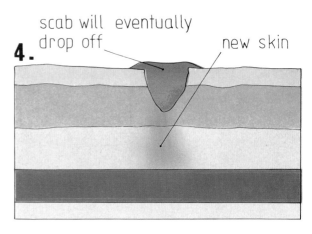

4. scab will eventually drop off   new skin

Under the scab the cut mends. When the cut has mended, the scab dries up and drops off.

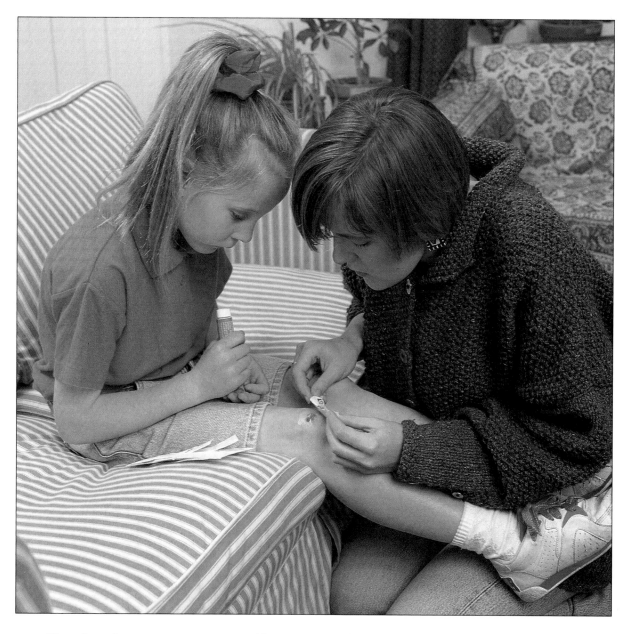

▲ To help stop a cut becoming infected, you must make sure it is clean. Wash it with clean water and then use antiseptic cream and a sticking plaster. Never pick a scab as it can open the cut again.

Infections

If dirt gets into a cut and your blood can't fight the infection, then the cut goes septic. This means the number of germs has grown. This can damage your skin or even make you ill.

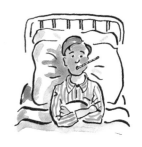

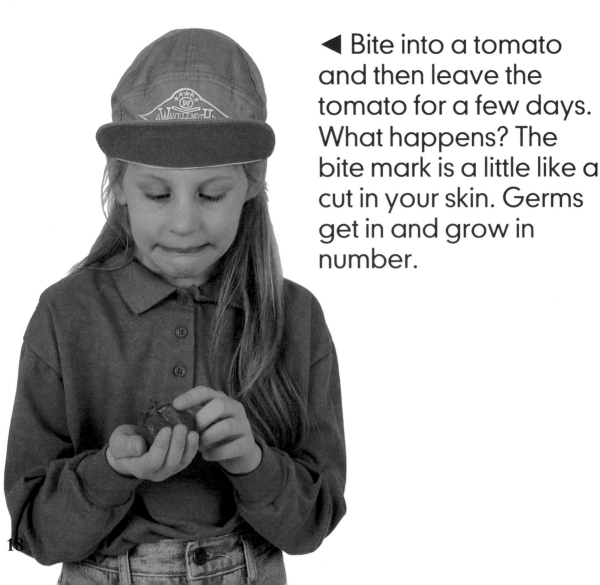

◀ Bite into a tomato and then leave the tomato for a few days. What happens? The bite mark is a little like a cut in your skin. Germs get in and grow in number.

If you cut yourself badly, you may need a tetanus booster. This is an injection which helps your blood to fight a nasty infection called tetanus. ▼

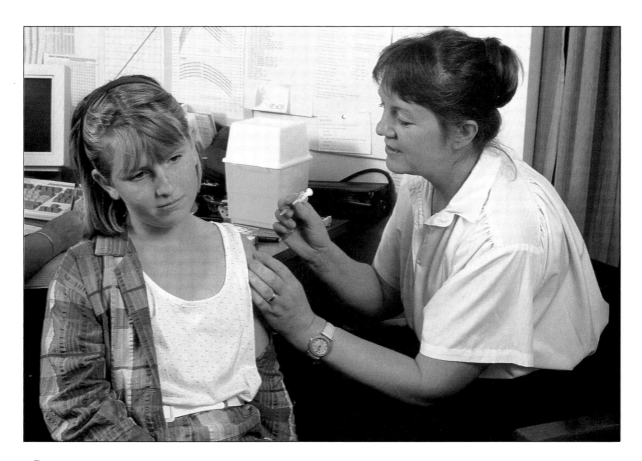

One very dangerous illness is AIDS. It can be caught if blood from a person with AIDS gets into someone else's open cut. Dentists wear thin rubber gloves to protect them from any small cuts they might get from teeth. You can't catch AIDS just by touching someone or by drinking from someone else's cup.

Clean hair

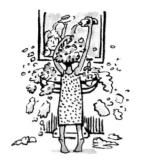

Lovely shiny hair means you are healthy and are eating the right things. If you are not eating the right food your hair can look dull.

Dirty hair will not let germs into your body, but it looks a mess.

Washing and rinsing your hair at least once a week keeps it clean.
▼

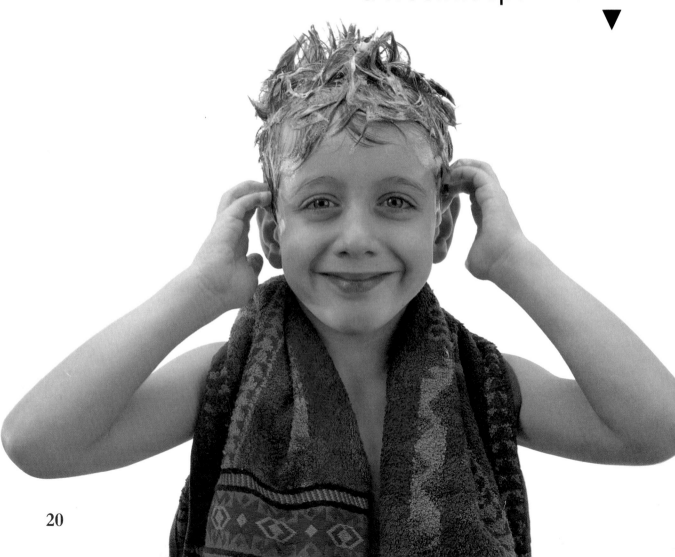

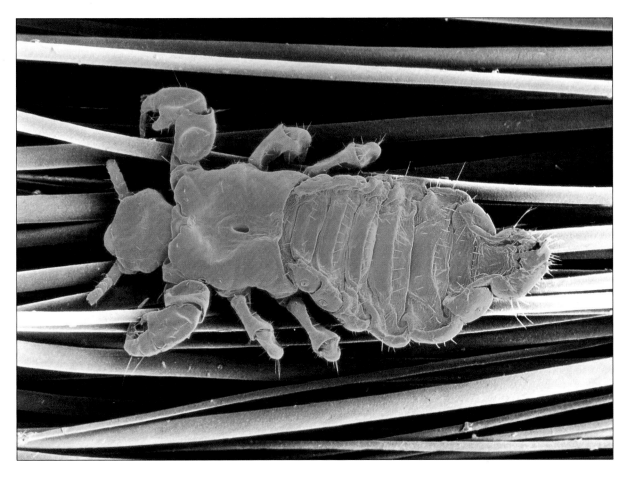

▲ Even clean hair can get head lice. This is what a head louse looks like under a microscope. False colour has been added. Head lice lay tiny white eggs called nits. To get rid of head lice you need a special shampoo and a very fine comb which pulls the lice and nits away from your hair.

WOW!
There are about 100,000 hairs on a person's head. Hair grows about 13 cm a year, but it only grows to about 80 cm long altogether.

Clean food

One way germs can get inside your body is through your mouth. You should always wash your hands after using the toilet to make sure any germs are washed away.

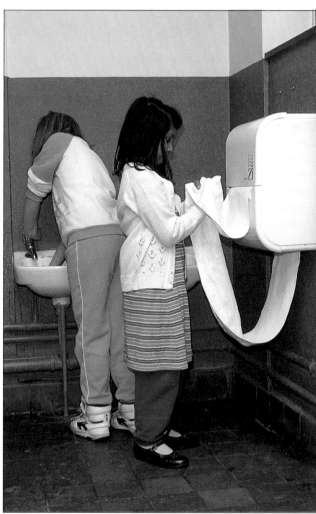

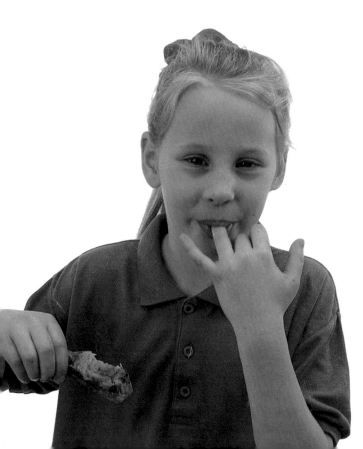

Also, you should wash your hands before you eat.

◄ Try not to lick dirty fingers!

Germs are always around us. If we let them grow and multiply they may harm us. Germs grow best in warm places. Food should be kept in a fridge and used before its sell-by-date.

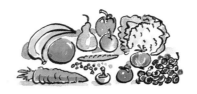

Look at the sell-by-dates or use-by-dates on different types of food at home. Which keep safe for a long time? Which don't? ▼

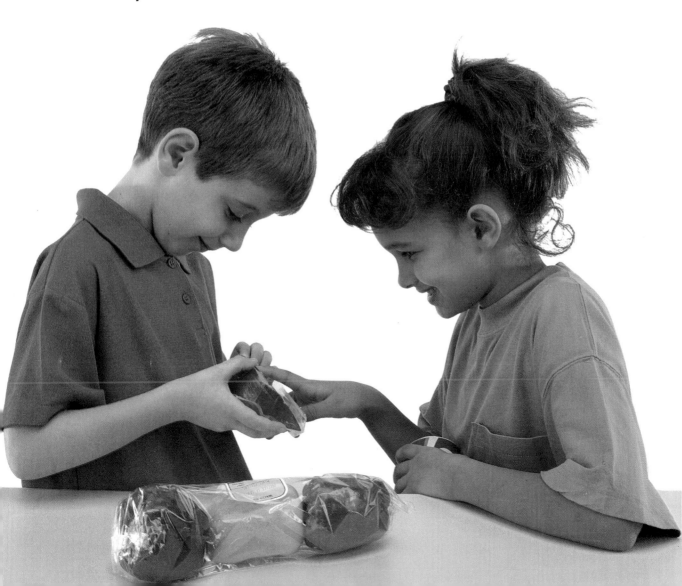

Clean water

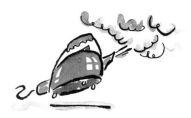

In most of Europe tap water is cleaned so it is fit to drink. But water can carry germs. Drinking dirty water allows germs to get inside us and make us ill. ▼

If water is not clean the best thing to do is boil it. This will kill most of the germs. But remember, never boil a kettle unless an adult is with you.

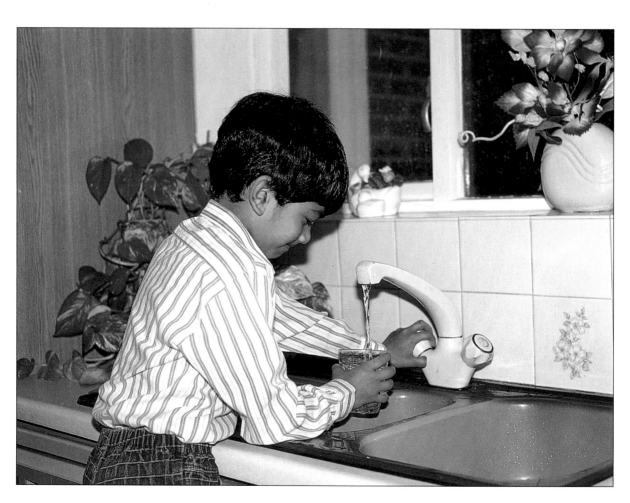

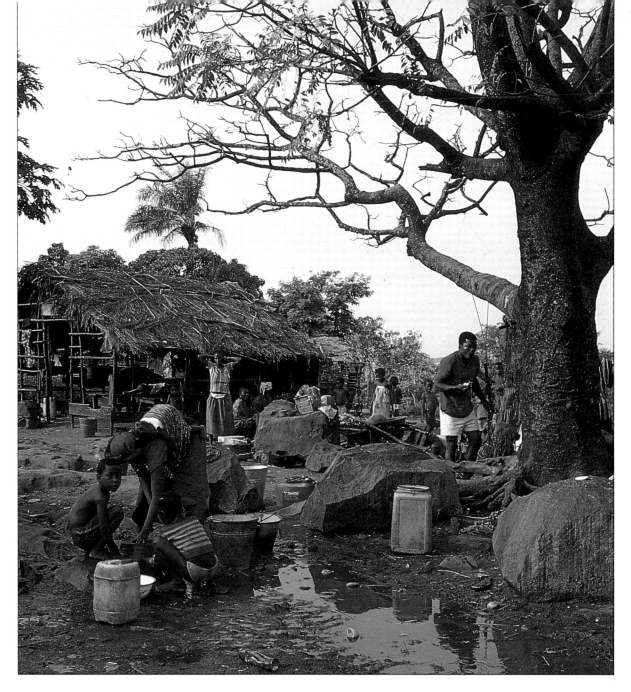

Water is precious. We all need it to live. Many people who live in hot dry countries die because they don't have fresh clean water.

Coughs and sneezes

Coughs and sneezes spread diseases.

You sneeze when the hairs up your nose are tickled. Your sneeze blows away the cause of the itch.

When you sneeze, tiny droplets escape into the air. These can contain germs which can be breathed in by somebody else. So always sneeze into a handkerchief. ▼

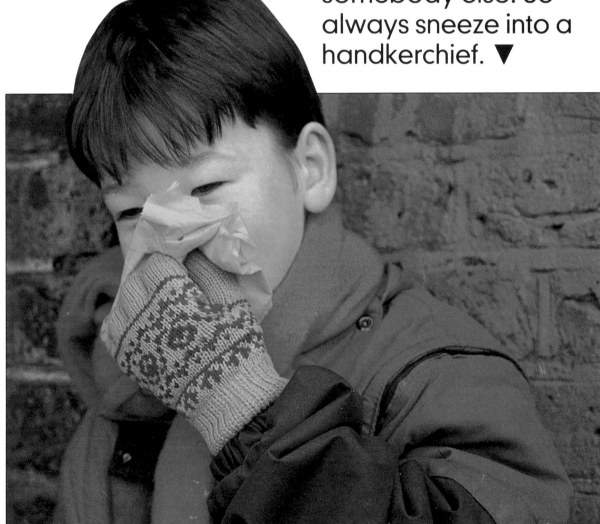

Most children in Britain now have an injection to stop them from getting measles, mumps and German measles, but the germs can be spread by coughing. This is why you should keep away from other children when you are ill. Don't pass on your germs!

name	'flu	measles	mumps	German measles	T. B.	Scarlet fever
Susan	✓					
Mr Johns	✓		✓	✓		
Grandma	✓	✓	✓	✓	✓	✓

▲ Which illnesses have you or your friends had? Which have your parents, grandparents or teachers had? Are there any illnesses that seem to have disappeared? If you copy this chart, it will help you with your investigations.

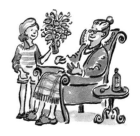

Fighting infection

Resistance is how well your body can fight germs. Some people can't fight infection as easily as others. Their resistance is poor.

A newborn baby's body hasn't learnt how to fight germs yet. It has to be kept very clean. This little girl has just had a bath. ▼

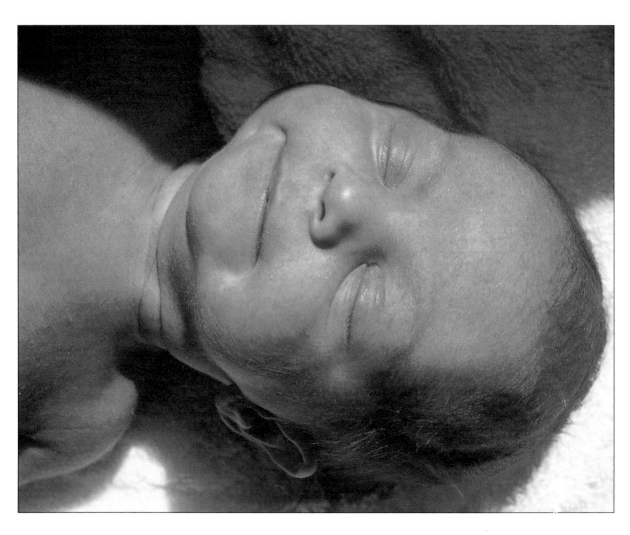

When someone is recovering from an illness they may have less strength to fight infection. Old people, in particular, can become ill quite easily. ▼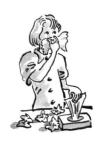

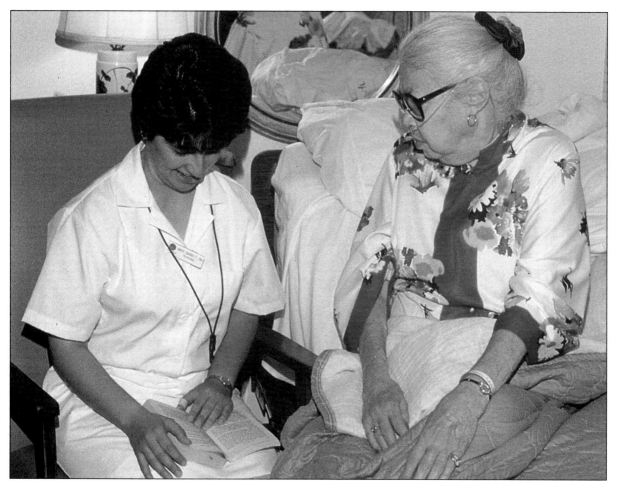

People who cannot get clean water or do not have enough to eat also have less resistance to infection.

Glossary

AIDS   A dangerous illness which can make a person's body unable to fight even small infections.

Antiseptic   A cream or liquid that kills germs.

Bacteria   A type of germ.

Disclosing tablets   Tablets used to show up plaque on teeth. The tablets dye the teeth where plaque has formed.

Diseases   Illnesses. Chicken Pox is a disease; a cold is another type of disease.

Fungus   A type of germ.

Head lice   Small creatures that live in hair.

Infections   Illnesses or sores caused by germs. We catch an infection when we catch a cold. We have an infected cut if it goes septic.

Measles   A common children's illness. It is not usually serious in Europe. But measles kills hundreds of children, especially in poor countries.

Nits   The eggs laid by head lice. They are white and stick to the hair.

Plaque   A thin sticky coating of bacteria on teeth.

Septic   Infected with germs. If a cut has gone septic you can see yellow pus in the cut. This means that bacteria have got into the cut and have increased in number.

Tetanus   A serious infection caused by certain bacteria entering a cut and getting into the blood.

Virus   A very small germ which can cause illness.

Books to read

There are lots of ideas in this book that you may want to explore further. Here are some books for you to read:

The Getting Better Book by Claire Rayner (Pan Books, 1986)
Health and Hygiene by Dorothy Baldwin (Wayland, 1990)
Going to the Dentist by K. Petty & L. Kopper (Franklin Watts, 1988)
The Tale of Mucky Mabel by J. Willis & M. Chamberlain (Arrow Books, 1984)

Index